Triplet Pregnancy

And Your First Year With Triplets

By N. T. Gore

Table of Contents

The Joy of Triplets

Congratulations on your triplet pregnancy! In the U.S. in the year 2000, there were 6,740 triplet births. In the natural course of things, the odds of spontaneously conceiving triplets are somewhere around 1 in 8,100, but these days, only about 30% of triplet pregnancies are natural, or "spontaneous" in origin.

Most triplet pregnancies these days are the result of fertility treatment, but you have a greater chance of spontaneously conceiving twins if you are African-American, an older mom, or have a family history of multiple births.

Either way, congratulate yourself. Whether it's been a long, hard road to conceive or this has all come as a big, fat surprise, you're on the way to being a mom in a whole different way from what you might have had planned.

Let's get started on the journey together.

How you'll feel at first.

If you conceived as a result of fertility treatment, you may have known you were expecting triplets right from the start.

That doesn't mean you're any less blown away by the news!

Bringing one new life into the world can be an overwhelming feeling... let alone three.

Katie: "OMG, I'm pregnant with triplets! Of course, I was on Clomid for 2 months, the lowest dose of 50mg, so it's not the biggest surprise. I guess it worked!"

Christine: "I am 8 weeks, 4 days along with triplets, so it's still early days. We've already seen heart beats for all three and they're in different sacs, as far as my doc can tell. Our triplets are natural, no drugs or any other treatments... but that's not what everybody will assume."

Maybe you found out a bit later in your pregnancy than other triplet moms. It's rare, but it *can* happen that one of the three was "hiding" behind the others and be missed on early ultrasounds.

Your practitioner may have been surprised by a third heartbeat during a regular checkup, or perhaps it was just discovered on a later ultrasound.

If that's you, you'll have a bit less time to adjust to the news than other triplet moms, who can find out these days as early as eight or ten weeks along.

Another kind of triplet mom is one who was originally expecting more babies – quads or quintuplets – whose pregnancy was either reduced by her doctor or who lost one or more fetuses.

If that's you, you'll have to mourn the lost pregnancy while finding enough love to embrace the three you are actually going to get to meet in person.

No matter when and how you found out, you'll probably be in shock – possibly for the duration of your pregnancy. It's a lot to think about!

This book will help you look at the realities in a way that isn't too technical or scary and to understand a little bit about the road that lies ahead.

Tina: My husband and I took a while to get used to the idea. The first week was the hardest. You'll probably go through some big swings, but that's normal: all those hormones plus life-shattering news will do that to you!

Proceed with caution.

It's tragic, but true. With the increased risks to each baby as a result of their cohabitation, and the greater chance of complications, many pregnancies that start out with triplets end up being born as twins or even singleton births.

> Louisa: "I originally had triplets, but one sac didn't have a heart and didn't develop as the others did. We're currently 20 weeks along with twins we can't wait to meet."

> Jacqui: "With these triplets, a scan put me at 6 weeks, but they've only seen one heartbeat so far. One sac looks empty, and they couldn't tell with the other one."

> Tessa: "Yesterday, we saw three healthy babies measuring big for their age! I am so excited but I've had two miscarriages, so we're naturally feeling nervous, too."

Sometimes, one fetus is lost early on and it's impossible to know why. In other cases, particularly farther along, it's easier to tell what went wrong.

But it's always difficult to lose a baby, especially after you've already adjusted – on some level – to the massive changes that a triplet parent, and being a triplet parent, will demand from you.

But it's also true that some moms may feel a bit relieved when they've lost one or more babies from a triplet pregnancy, particularly if they were lost early on (a late-term loss is a lot more traumatic and takes a greater physical toll as well). Triplets are a lot to take on! Of course, those moms were prepared to look after three babies if they had to, but if one is lost naturally, they realize the task ahead may be a bit easier.

Even if you're secretly hoping, on some level, that one of the babies will be lost, that doesn't make you a monster. This is all part of the normal mix of feelings when you're waiting for triplets.

Siobhan: "Don't lose hope! Last week, at six weeks, we saw only one heartbeat. I was so sad. Today, exactly one week later, we saw three strong heartbeats!"

Selective Reduction

It's not as common with triplets as it is with quads and beyond, but if you have health problems or special risks, your practitioner may recommend "selectively reducing" the pregnancy.

This is an abortion, performed very early on, which will generally target the least viable baby – perhaps due to concerns about blood supply or slow development.

Sarah: "I'm 29 and conceived through IVF. I'm on the petite side, 5'1" and 107 pounds before I got pregnant. My doctor is trying to persuade me to 'selectively reduce' one of these babies for my own safety as well as to protect the other two, but I don't know what to do."

With a decision this big, it's worth getting a second opinion, since views on the viability of the babies may vary.

There are risks associated with reduction, as well, and doctors are still uncertain if the risks of carrying triplets to term outweigh those of reducing the pregnancy. Even if everyone agrees that it must be done, you'll be relieved knowing there really was no choice.

Why it's not as scary as you think.

Allison: "I was terrified, confused, you name it, it was such a mind-blowing time. I'd say it wasn't until twenty-plus weeks before I came to terms with it all. Maybe a few weeks before my kiddoes were born… and then I was just so, so excited to meet them."

We've all heard the expression, "God never gives you a job you can't handle."

Parents of triplets discover within themselves unknown, untapped reserves of energy, resourcefulness and love that they never thought themselves capable of before.

Sure, you'll get overwhelmed – who wouldn't, at the prospect of three new mouths to feed, bottoms pooping and everything in between.

But you will enjoy so much love, more than you could ever have imagined, over the years to come.

Your home will be full (okay, sometimes too full) of noise and laughter. Before we get into the nitty-gritty, let's explore why you're going to love having that houseful of noise.

What you'll LOVE about triplets!

Laura: "Triplets are intense in every way. Sure, you'll feel overwhelmed, but then there are days when you'll feel overwhelmed with love. We wouldn't trade those days for anything in the world."

Most parents of triplets love the unique experience it offers their kids growing up. They'll never be lonely, they'll have constant companionship at least through the first part of their lives. Sure, they'll probably keep secrets from you, almost from their very first days at home, but they'll also surprise you with their sweetness, day after day.

If you came from a big family, you'll probably love the feeling of having your house full, and recreating the big-family dynamics you enjoyed as a kid... all in one pregnancy.

If you didn't, it may take a little adjusting, unless you were one of those children who always envied the big, busy families on your block.

You'll love discovering that you can still be you, even if you have to adjust the way you do things a little. If you're a neat freak, you can still be a neat freak, and after you get into a routine with the babies, this orderliness can help them immensely.

On the other hand, if your style is more casual and love spontaneous family outings, you'll naturally have three willing accomplices to go along for the ride.

You will be raising your babies your way, but you'll also love watching yourself proudly accomplishing things that would have seemed impossible a year or two before.

Your friends will watch in admiration, even if that admiration takes the form of headshaking and muttering that they could never do the things you do. If they had triplets, they'd do it all too.

You'll love the days when you conquer the mess and clutter and everybody goes to bed happy.

On all the other days, you'll remember the challenge involved and forgive yourself to start fresh again in the morning.

What you'll HATE about triplets!

Sandra: "Let yourself mourn the experience you might have wanted. It's okay to be disappointed even if everybody tells you how happy you should feel. But then regroup and figure out what's most important (about the birth and parenting), and what you can do to get as much of that as you can."

If you went through fertility treatment, everybody may assume you're thrilled now that you have triplets on the way.

You'll never need to try to conceive again! Your family will be complete all in one pregnancy!

But that's probably not how you envisioned becoming a parent (if this is your first time) or having your next baby (if you've already had kids).

It's okay to mourn the experience you wanted – to say, this isn't ideal, this isn't what everybody else is doing, and I wanted something a little more normal.

Julie: "I'm 24 weeks now, but it took me a few weeks early on to mourn the implications... my small family was no longer going to be anywhere near small, ever again. I'm still not sure I'm totally at peace with all this will mean for us, but I think I'm getting close."

It's also okay to look at the things you're sure to hate about triplet pregnancy and life with triplets at home, especially during the first year.

During the pregnancy, you'll hate what's happening to your body and the loss of control you'll feel – even if you've been pregnant before, because this pregnancy is different from anything you've ever experienced (and probably from anything your friends and family have been through, too!).

Once the babies are home, you will never have enough hands, and you may never feel competent enough to deal with the incessant needs of all those babies.

You'll hate the loss of sleep and you may well hate your partner or spouse and even blame him for getting you here in the first place.

Hate is a strong word, but it's a word that *will* bubble up into your brain over months to come. Don't be afraid of it. Of course, you should try to look on the bright side, but glossing over hard times never fixed anything.

Find good friends you can talk to, and maybe even a professional if things seem too overwhelming.

First Steps

We're expecting triplets – what should we do?

Michelle: "Congratulate yourself! I bet you're still in shock. Hey, I'm still in shock and my babies are almost a year old. I think I'll probably be in some form of shock for the rest of my life. Things can go really well with a triplet pregnancy, so don't get discouraged. Stay positive and keep eating for your own strength. It's been fun so far – if more intense than I ever bargained on."

Sit down. Take a deep breath. You probably don't have to do anything right away.

Good, now that that's done, your feelings may be mixed. You may want to jump up and run around and scream in triumph that you're pregnant at last – and how! Or, honestly, you may just want to throw up and crawl back into bed. Both of those reactions are normal.

Lacey: "We were so, so very shocked at our first ultrasound, and still go through waves of 'OMG!' The logistics are staggering! I have two kids already, but feel like a first-time mom all over again at pregnancy number three!"

Ultimately, you're going to need to get your act together to prepare for a triplet pregnancy, which is like nothing you've ever experienced before.

You'll need to choose a practitioner very early on, and your pregnancy will most likely be classified as "high risk," which means you won't have a lot of choices about who takes care of you during pregnancy.

Whoever you pick will fill you in on any health precautions you'll need to know about. If you haven't seen anyone yet, you should start taking a supplement with folic acid, if you weren't already when trying to conceive.

And whatever you do, you'll need to tell your family and friends. That can be a fun adventure all by itself.

Breaking the News

As with any pregnancy, your family and friends want to know your news, and everybody wants to be the first to hear. This can be tricky territory. You may well be closer to your mom than to your mother-in-law (most women are), but your mother-in-law could be tremendously hurt if you tell your mother as soon as you get that positive pregnancy test... and then only tell her when you're starting to show.

With triplets, there are two stages to breaking the news: revealing that you're pregnant... and revealing that it's not one, not two, but three little ones you're preparing for.

If there's any doubt about the viability of one or more babies, you might want to hold off telling anybody you're expecting triplets.

Some women don't even reveal that they're pregnant until after the risky first semester has passed. On the other hand, since you're expecting triplets, you will probably show very early and appear very large for your dates. So people may catch on quickly and then feel hurt that you didn't tell them.

Ultimately, you and your partner should decide when's the right time to reveal both of these pieces of information, and to whom. Don't tell anyone you're not comfortable telling! Worst case scenario, they'll probably figure it out for themselves sooner or later (with triplets, more likely sooner than later).

If you have kids already, knowing when to tell them is always tricky. Most kids don't understand the greater risk of miscarriage in the first trimester, so if you tell them there's going to be a baby, that's what they'll expect.

They may be devastated if anything happens to one or more babies. But there's another hand, too: most big siblings like to feel involved with the pregnancy. And, of course, because of the physical toll triplet pregnancy can take at any time, you'll probably need whatever help the big sibs can offer.

At work, you may need to break the news of your pregnancy earlier than you'd like, for example, if you're experiencing spotting and need to stay home on bed rest for a few days.

That doesn't mean you have to subject yourself to the office gossip mill: tell one or two people who need to know, in confidence, and ask them not to share this information. You can even tell them it's because you're worried you may lose one or more babies. Generally, they'll respect this request.

Choosing a Practitioner

Don't be alarmed when you find out that almost all multiple pregnancies these days are classed as "high-risk." That doesn't automatically mean your babies are at risk! It just means that you'll need to choose a specialist practitioner, most likely an OB-Gyn who handles pregnancies like this as the majority of his or her practice.

It's very unlikely that you'll find a midwife or nurse-midwife who's able to take on your care as your main practitioner.

One possibility, if you're looking for a more holistic approach to pregnancy care than the sterile setting of an OB's office can provide, is to find a doula who can help you with your pregnancy, birth, and homecoming. Be certain that wherever your doctor delivers allows doulas in the operating room during C-sections.

Some hospitals have been resistant to doulas, even though their use generally improves outcomes for moms and babies even when surgery is inevitable.

If you're outside of a major metropolitan area, your practitioner may have a more generalized practice, not limited to high-risk or multiple pregnancies. Make sure early on that he or she has sufficient connections to transfer you and/or your babies to a "tertiary," or more advanced facility in the nearest urban area at the first sign of trouble. Talk this over at your first visits and write down the answers – where you or the babies would be transferred to (there may be a separate children's hospital) and how the transfer would take place (ambulance, helicopter), and under what circumstances this might happen.

Health Precautions

It's unanimous – start drinking now and don't stop until your triplets graduate from college. Okay, maybe not so long, but your water intake is one of the best ways to stay as strong and vigorous as possible.

With your own blood circulating among so many little ones, your blood pressure is almost certain to drop and with it, your energy levels. Drinking water makes sure there's enough to go around.

Tina: That first trimester may be rough. Treat yourself as gently as possible, and I'd say go with whatever you're feeling and craving. I tried to focus on getting enough protein and calcium, and kept an eye on my weight gain. That way, even if things get out of control later on, I felt like I had a solid foundation.

Other than eating and drinking properly from the start, there aren't necessarily many health precautions for early on in a triplet pregnancy. In fact, most triplet moms can do anything they'd normally do, albeit at a slower pace and resting more often.

If you conceived through fertility treatment, your doctor may let you know about hormones and other supplements that you'll need to keep taking throughout early pregnancy. And your doctor may also have something to say on the issue of sex. Check to see if it's allowed throughout the pregnancy or will be restricted at some point.

Preparing for the Pregnancy

Finding out you're expecting triplets can come as a major blow if you were hoping for a more holistic approach to pregnancy.

Plenty of triplet moms come into the triplet experience after a very "natural" first pregnancy in which they may have given birth at home with a midwife, cloth-diapered, breastfed, teethed on organic foods only, and more.

Some of those things may still be possible with triplets – but others won't be.

Bailey: "What the first year looks like depends a lot on how well you and the babies handle the pregnancy and how much help you have. If you carry close to term and have lots of help and the babies are happy and healthy, you may be able to do everything you dream of, whether that's breastfeeding, cosleeping, however you see yourself raising these babies. On the other hand, if you or the babies develop complications, you may need to rethink those priorities in light of your new reality. I'd say be flexible and enjoy the wildest ride of your life."

Beyond emotional preparations, and getting over the fact that this may not be the pregnancy you'd dreamed of, you'll want to get ready in sort of the same way you'd get ready for a trip to a new and fascinating country: learning the language, as well as all about the customs, food and clothing of that country. Welcome to the land of triplet pregnancy!

Learn the Lingo: A quick glossary

Placentas / Sacs: What's the difference?

Triplet pregnancies are generally classified according to both how many placentas there are and how many amniotic sacs have been developed to hold the babies.

In general, there's a higher risk when multiple babies are sharing a placenta. The most common result is what's often known as "twin-to-twin transfer syndrome" or TTTS, which is more accurately called Feto-fetal transfusion syndrome when it occurs in triplet or higher pregnancies.

Chorionic = how many placentas there are	Amniotic = how many sacs there are
Monochorionic one placenta (all babies share the placenta)	Monoamniotic one sac holds all 3 babies (only one placenta)
Dichorionic two placentas (two babies share one placenta)	Diamniotic two sacs (may be one or two placentas)

Trichorionic	Triamniotic
three placentas	three sacs (may be one, two or three placentas)

Are they identical?

Be prepared: the first question people may ask is, "are they identical?" Sure, identical triplets are possible, caused by a single fertilized egg splitting into three babies, but this is really rare, maybe occurring in less than 6% of natural triplet pregnancies.

More often, the babies are fraternal, meaning they don't look more alike than any other brothers and sisters, but it is possible to have a combination of two identical twins with the third baby related to the others fraternally. If your babies aren't all the same sex, there's no chance that they're identical.

An early ultrasound may be able to detect that all three babies are sharing the same placenta and sac. If that's the case, they may be able to tell you your babies are identical.

Another method is to inspect the placenta and sacs after birth, but even this isn't always conclusive.

Short of DNA testing, there are no other ways to tell whether your triplets are genetically identical, even if they look very similar... but you'll probably discover soon enough that they're not.

Other helpful terminology

B, G, BGG, BBG, etc.	B and G are short for "boy" and "girl". These 3-letter codes tell everybody what combination of triplets you're expecting.
Fraternal	Triplets who resemble each other only as much as ordinary siblings would.
Identical	Genetically the same in every way – can be verified only with DNA testing.
IVF	In-vitro fertilization.
IUI	Intra-uterine insemination.
Reduction	Using a modified abortion procedure to "cull" an unhealthy, undersized or otherwise non-viable fetus.
Spontaneous	Sometimes called "natural" – when triplets or higher-order multiples are conceived without fertility treatment.
Tertiary Center	Regional hospital with experienced expert staff and

	facilities for complicated pregnancies and neonatal ICU facilities to care for premature babies.
Zygosity	A zygote is the combination of egg and sperm we all learned about in health class. Triplet pregnancies can be monozygotic (identical), dizygotic (one zygote splits to include a set of identical twins), or – most commonly – trizygotic, or fraternal.
MFM	Maternal-fetal medicine, a practitioner or practice that specializes in care for high-risk pregnancies.

Special Challenges

Patricia: "I'm 31 weeks along with my triplets. I've been blessed with a complication-free pregnancy so far, but I know I'm lucky. Even without complications, it's exhausting, so take super care of yourself. Rest as much as you can, eat lots to grow those babies nice and big. And like everybody else will probably tell you: water, water, water... drink it until you burst!"

Take all the challenges of a singleton pregnancy... and multiple them by three. Then double them. And double them again. You will reach a point in your pregnancy when you believe the human body wasn't engineered to take this kind of strain, and you'll be half-right.

There's a reason triplet pregnancy is so rare in nature – it really is pushing the limits of what we're capable of doing.

But you can get through it and stay healthy, which is not to say that you'll be free of aches and pains. The strain on your body is real, and because you're going to be so much bigger and heavier than a woman with a singleton pregnancy, you're going to be putting all that much more stress on your joints, ligaments and other tender regions.

These stresses will also arrive earlier in pregnancy than they would with just one baby. Most women with a single pregnancy can eat reasonably normally until the last trimester, for example, when the baby starts crowding out their stomach.

Sorry – your three babies are going to be clamoring for space a lot sooner than that, meaning all the unpleasant side-effects like heartburn and reduced appetite, at a time when you need to be eating better than ever.

Later on in pregnancy, you'll be at higher risk for preterm labor, preeclampsia and gestational diabetes.

But that doesn't mean you're off the hook for more mundane problems, experienced by all moms, like morning sickness, maternity clothing, choosing a balanced diet, keeping up your sexuality, and more.

Morning Sickness

You've already heard by now – it's not just in the morning, it can last all day, all night, and yes, even all through your pregnancy. And it's no joke, despite an early-morning bathroom run being the way that most women in movies (especially comedies) find out they're expecting.

Thought to be a reaction to the wash of chemicals flooding your body in the first trimester, that explains why it can plague moms of triplets even when they've never experienced a minute of morning sickness in other pregnancies.

For most women, morning sickness eases by the end of the first trimester. This is sometimes the case with triplet pregnancies as well, as your body acclimatizes to the hormonal onslaught and things balance out a little.

But be prepared for the possibility that it may not go away at all. If nausea becomes a more serious problem and you're not able to take in enough nutrition, you may be suffering from hyperemesis gravidarum, a serious condition – please see your doctor.

Fashion

What to wear when you're expecting has probably been on the forefront of pregnant moms' minds since the fall of the Roman empire and the demise of the toga.

In your case, you probably won't find the clothes you need in any kind of maternity clothing store – most of those clothes barely fit normal women all the way through a standard pregnancy!

You may be able to find secondhand clothing that fits comfortably by networking with other multiple moms who have a few precious pieces that took them all the way through.

In general, it's best to put fashion on the back burner for a few months, with the attitude that this is all temporary – you may well be right back to wearing your skinny jeans in just a few months after the babies arrive.

It's worth mentioning here that whatever you've heard about foot size may in fact be true – many women gain a whole shoe size during pregnancy, so you may need to shop for a whole new shoe wardrobe.

It probably won't be fun, either, considering you won't be able to see your feet all that well.

Choose shoes for comfort and durability rather than fashion at this point. Feet also rarely go back to the same size after pregnancy, so pick shoes that will last, and consider getting rid of some of the more impractical selections in your wardrobe.

Diet

Shira: *"We all left the hospital together after only five days; the boys didn't spend even a minute in the NICU. I really think I carried so long and the boys were such good weights, so healthy, because of my highly disciplined diet. It wasn't easy: I forced myself to eating healthy, no cheating. But now I know it was so worth it!"*

Every calorie counts, in any pregnancy, but even more so in a triplet pregnancy. Most experienced moms will tell you to eat any healthy food you can take. Keeping up a great diet is a challenge for different reasons at different points in your pregnancy.

In early pregnancy, morning sickness can get in the way, so finding foods that don't nauseate you can be tough. When you do, stick with them – don't worry about the carbs in the soda crackers if they're the only thing you can keep down!

Later on (usually the third trimester for one-baby pregnancies, but usually the second for triplets), eating is hard simply because there's not enough space in your abdomen (no matter how it expands!) for three babies plus a full big meal.

Greasy foods – or any food – may give you heartburn or worse.

At this point, you'll need to switch to small meals, and eat more often to give yourself the energy boost you'll need.

Guidelines for a twin pregnancy generally suggest eating an extra 500 calories a day, which is calculated based on 300 for the first baby (what you'd eat if you only had one in there), plus 200 for each baby after that.

So with triplets on the way, you'll need even more: probably around 700 calories extra. Of course, you should also continue taking prenatal vitamins once they've been okayed by your doctor.

A word of caution about supplements and teas: Certain herbal supplements and teas are associated with preterm labor, so you will want to discuss everything you're taking with your doctor, even if it's "all natural." Remember, poison ivy and hemlock are all-natural, too!

Comfort

Oh, the aches and pains of childbearing! Some will come and go... and others will just drop in and stay, perhaps for life.

Round ligament pain

The round ligament connects your uterus to your pelvis, so that's where you're likely to feel discomfort – even in a standard pregnancy, this is one of the most common aches and pains. Pain in this area is felt as a sharp or jabbing pain in the lower belly and groin.

Lots of things can bring it on, including sneezing, coughing, sudden position changes, or – sadly – laughing too much or too hard. Because it comes on so quickly, you may feel like something is wrong with you or your pregnancy.

Round ligament pain can also be confused with preterm contractions, so it's best to report it to your practitioner. But most often, after checking carefully, you'll be reassured to know it's normal.

Avoiding round ligament pain completely is probably impossible in a triplet pregnancy, but keeping your core and back muscles strong with prenatal exercise (as long as you can keep it up comfortably and safely) can help avoid the worst of it.

You may also find some positions that make it more comfortable to cough, sneeze and laugh.

Round ligament pain can be treated over-the-counter pain relief once your doctor okays it, and applying warmth to the region can also be helpful – again, with your practitioner's permission.

Sciatica

Here's another one of those aches and pains that, for most women, shows up late in pregnancy, but which you may start experiencing as early as nine to twelve weeks. Sciatica is pain caused by compression of one or the other sciatic nerves, which run from the lower back down into your legs.

During pregnancy, it's normal for the baby to press down on this nerve, which can cause back and leg pain ranging from mild to severe. It can also numb your legs, making it hard to balance.

There's not much anyone can do about sciatica, other than moving around to encourage the babies to change position and get off those nerves!

Balance

Many women experience balance problems during pregnancy, and there are a couple of causes, including dizziness and low blood pressure due to increased blood volume, along with – of course – the changing shape of their body.

As with every other symptom, both of these issues are greatly increased in a triplet pregnancy, and you'll probably find it difficult to balance through most or at least part of your pregnancy. Be extra careful!

Sometimes, a shift in the babies' positions will shift your center of balance just enough that your body doesn't behave as you expect it to, which can lead to dangerous falls.

Other aches, pains and irritations

Melody: "I'm 25 weeks along now, and I get horribly dizzy when I have to lie on my back. I don't know how I'm going to make it through all those ultrasounds! And it's hard to sleep. I get up about every 4 hours to pee and drink more water, but I'm waking up a lot more because every time I change position it hurts. Let's not forget **the Braxton-Hicks contractions! But I am so glad I'm not on bed rest... and my cervix is still long and closed.**"

It's an old joke, but it's true. If any one of these symptoms was happening to a guy, whether it was too-frequent urination, dizziness, crippling nausea or stabbing back or stomach pains, he'd run screaming to the E.R.

But for the rest of us, who are creating new life and bringing it into the world three times over, we just have to bear with it and hope it will all be over soon – which it usually is. Your hips and feet will hurt when you walk; your back and hips will hurt when you sit or lie down… and by the way, it will be nearly impossible to get back up again once you do. That doesn't mean you should ignore every new symptom!

Especially if an unfamiliar pain or intense sensation comes on quickly, you should let your practitioner know what's going on. Chances are, there's little he or she can do, but keeping a vigilant watch over your own body will make sure nothing more serious is going on.

Useful tools

At some point, if you're having a lot of discomfort, your practitioner may recommend some form of orthopedic support – something to help your back and stomach muscles handle the tremendous burden that's being put on them.

A back or front support (one popular model is the "Prenatal Cradle") can be a great way to physically hold up your growing belly and take pressure off your back muscles as well as the round ligaments.

Mindy: "It helped a lot when I was up and about – it helped stop the feeling that my belly was going to fall off. I actually went through two because I outgrew the first one!"

A visit to a surgical supply store may pay off in terms of some other useful tools to manage the last weeks of pregnancy and the first few weeks postpartum.

One of these is a "reach extender," which basically looks like a kid's toy you might use to grab things you can't reach.

They're sold for post-surgical patients who can't bend easily to pick things up off the floor or retrieve them from high places, and they can be the perfect thing for you as seeing (let alone touching) the floor becomes a distant, fond memory. (One company also makes a razor extender if you find you still want to keep your legs looking shiny and stubble-free!)

Keep an open mind! You may find other types of aids that you can use – often they can be rented from medical-supply centers – to make life around your house more livable. These are products designed for older people and those with disabilities.

Particularly in the bathroom, some of these ingenious creations can greatly add to your ease and comfort during the last few weeks of pregnancy and even beyond, when you're recovering from what's likely to be a surgical delivery.

Think about getting safety bars in the shower and perhaps beside the toilet, and you may also want to consider a raised toilet seat. Sitting and standing, things we always take for granted, can be nearly impossible towards the end!

Don't be embarrassed that friends and family might see these tools when they come to visit – the important thing here is keeping you healthy and as comfortable as possible.

Another great tool: a swimming pool! Just spending a few minutes or more in the water can take away lots of the pressure you're body's experience and give you a brief respite of comfort in the middle of what can be an oppressive experience.

Bed Rest

Here it is... the dreaded "B-word" of any multiples pregnancy. The first thing to know is that it may never happen, but there's a good chance it will. There are so many possible reasons a mom could be "put on bed rest" at any point in her pregnancy, so you must be ready for this eventuality, even if it never happens.

If your doctor says you must go on bed rest, find out exactly what this means. The term actually refers to an entire spectrum that could include drastically reducing your physical activity (but not being literally confined to your bed 24/7), but still being able to get up and move around, or it could mean lying on your side all the time and even using a bedpan.

In most cases, getting up for short periods to use the bathroom or to shower is allowed.

Bed rest may sound like a much-needed break from daily life, but as anyone who's been there knows, it's truly a traumatic experience, physically, mentally and emotionally.

You'll need to call in all the support you can get to get you through this difficult, isolating, painful and – if your babies are in jeopardy – potentially frightening time.

Childcare

Even if you're not on bed rest, you'll probably be exhausted throughout the last few weeks (or months) of your pregnancy. That's normal – the new normal of all that extra strain on your body.

If you have young kids, they're still going to need you around, of course, but they may not realize exactly what you're capable of (and not) these days.

That's when it helps to have an extra body – a friend, an older neighbor, a teenage girl who lives nearby – who can come by and give you a hand at your kids' neediest time(s) of day, whether that's before school in the morning or between dinner and bedtime.

If you're around and not on bed rest, you can even rely on responsible younger children, maybe a friend's or neighbor's kids, such as pre-teens who get along well with your children and can distract them with games or corral them through tooth brushing and a bedtime story.

Kids this age often love the responsible feeling of looking after other children, and you're there in case anything goes wrong.

Sexuality

Alla: "For the first 4 months, I was too busy trying not to be sick to let hubby anywhere near my lady parts. Now I'm 32 weeks, and more concerned with getting babies out then letting hubby in."

You may be wondering how this pregnancy is going to affect your sex life. Every woman's body is different, but you may actually be feeling more desire than usual during your pregnancy.

Some women feel super-sexy early in pregnancy, emboldened by the liberating idea that – for once – they can do whatever they want and they won't get pregnant.

For others, sexiness peaks around the middle of pregnancy, once the terrors of morning sickness are past and before their body becomes too bulky to maneuver.

Believe it or not, others find the end of pregnancy, when their body is awash in oxytocin, known as the "love hormone," the sexiest point in the whole experience (even though the actual experience may be complicated by their new, bulky shape).

Unfortunately, some women experience pregnancy as great, long void of sexual feelings. Either they're too emotionally distracted by the pregnancy or the prospect of birth, afraid of hurting the baby (even when their doctor gives the all-clear), or simply "not in the mood," that can put stress both on them and their partner, straining the relationship at a time when it should be strengthened.

Whether you're in the mood or not, don't have sex without checking with your doctor, especially if you're still on fertility hormones like progesterone or have reason to believe there might be a problem with the pregnancy.

Scared to ask your doctor? Don't be. Remember that women routinely poop, fart, puke and more during a standard vaginal delivery: your O.B. really has seen and heard it all. Talking about pleasure and fun could even be a welcome distraction for both of you.

If there's a nurse in the doctor's practice you get along with, you can talk to her as well, but remember that the doctor's advice is law when it comes to keeping your babies safe.

Tonya: "We haven't had sex since 21 weeks. The last time, it gave me such strong contractions afterwards, I got really scared. My doctor said it was okay at first, but after I had those contractions, he said we had to stop."

Marta: "I'm only 6 weeks, 6 days, and my doctor said no sex at all until after they're born. My husband isn't happy, and I'm not exactly cool *with it either. One of the nurses said he was this conservative with all his patients, but I think this is ridiculous. No sex? At all?"*

Nitty Gritty in Triplet City

Seeing your practitioner

Each practitioner has his or her own guidelines for safely managing a multiple pregnancy, but in general, you'll see him or her less often in the beginning, progressing to very frequent visits at the end of pregnancy.

Schedule of visits / tests

- 1-12 weeks: if all is normal, you may see your doctor only once a month at this point
- 10-12 weeks: CVS / nuchal translucency tests, if you opt to have these done
- 13-25 weeks: you'll probably see your doctor twice a month to ensure that all is well
- 16-20 weeks: amniocentesis, if you opt to have this done
- 20 weeks: you'll probably receive ultrasounds at least monthly from here on out
- 25+ weeks: you may be visiting your doctor every week at this point
- 28 weeks: your doctor may wish to perform a non-stress test (NST) weekly to keep tabs
- 33 weeks: this is considered "full-term" for a triplet pregnancy – anything more is a bonus!

Sizes / weights during average pregnancy

In triplet pregnancies, there isn't really an "official" weight gain guideline, but you should expect to gain at least 35 to 55 pounds. If you were underweight before becoming pregnant, you may even gain more. During the final six months of pregnancy, you'll probably gain about two pounds a week.

Although there aren't really guidelines for how much you should lose or gain, your practitioner will be keeping an eye on your measurements mainly to make sure that you're not gaining at an alarming rate and that your growth hasn't slowed for any reason.

Key Pregnancy Milestones

- At 12 weeks, the end of the first trimester, the risk of miscarriage in most pregnancies decreases. Often, nausea and morning sickness will pass by then, too.
- At 24 weeks, babies reach the "threshold of viability." Despite serious problems, about 1/3 of babies born at this point survive to live normal lives.
- At 28 weeks, odds of viability go up even higher, with 90% of babies making it this far surviving, though lasting problems (including cerebral palsy and blindness) are still a threat.
- At 32 to 34 weeks, babies have an excellent chance of survival without major long-term complications, though their lungs might not be fully mature yet and they may have

digestive or other problems that require a NICU stay.

- Between 33 and 37 weeks, babies' lungs mature and there is an excellent chance that they will be born healthy. Due to their tiny size, however, most triplets do require a NICU stay of some length, even if they're born this far along.

Routine Tests

Many of the tests listed below are part of a standard pregnancy testing regimen. However, some tests that yield useful results in a singleton pregnancy may not be as relevant for multiples like triplets. Some, for instance, rely on testing the baby itself (such as nuchal translucency), which may be difficult with multiple babies.

Others test the amniotic fluid surrounding the baby, procedures which have both increasing difficulty and increasing risk, depending on the number of sacs and placentas, among other factors.

As you get closer to the end of your pregnancy, you'll probably start being tested more often, with non-stress tests, biophysical profiles and tests like amniocentesis, which can tell you how ready the babies' lungs are for the stress of breathing on their own.

Rh Factor

This is one of the first tests of pregnancy. Most people are Rh positive, which means there's a common protein in their blood cells. If you lack this protein, there's a chance your baby could still have it – inherited from the father. If that's the case, your blood types are "incompatible," and your body may attack the "foreign" protein in the baby, causing anemia. In the past, this often led to infant death, but today, all Rh-negative mothers receive a series of injections which prevents this from happening. Rh incompatibility is generally not a problem as long as it's prevented in time.

Chorionic Villus Sampling (CVS) & Amniocentesis

These tests share many similarities. Both types of test require breaching the cozy environment of the womb in order to take samples that can reveal a lot of information about the wellbeing of the babies. Both tests can raise red flags about Down Syndrome, Tay-Sachs, hemophilia and other potential genetic problems. And both – naturally – are trickier if you're expecting twins than in a singleton pregnancy.

It's important to know that both tests are optional. Often, the information you receive may be confusing (warning of a potential problem that can't be resolved before delivery) or cause emotional conflict (uncertainty about whether to abort or reduce the pregnancy if one of the babies has a problem).

Before any test, you should find out what you're testing for and discuss with your partner what you will do with the information you receive. Hopefully, all will be well, but find out what the potential negative results are so you can deal with them just in case.

Both CVS and amniocentesis carry a risk of miscarriage, about 4%. In the hands of an experienced practitioner, the risk is about the same for each test.

CVS is often blamed for more miscarriages, but this is probably just a coincidence, because CVS is done during a higher-risk stage of pregnancy.

CVS is generally done earlier, between 10-12 weeks. A doctor enters your uterus, either through your abdomen or through your cervix, and draws a sample of the chorionic villus, tiny cells found in the placenta, which exactly mirror the genetic material in the baby's cells.

Amniocentesis, done between 15-20 weeks, uses the same principle, but studies the amniotic fluid instead, which contains loose cells that are tested for genetic and other disorders. Amniocentesis can also be done later to help determine how mature each baby's lungs are, which is crucial for determining if it's safe for them to be born.

Nuchal Translucency (NT)

This is another early test, done with an ultrasound, usually at the same time as CVS, since the data are often used together, along with blood test results, to create a picture of your babies' wellbeing. It is non-invasive; the technician measures the size of the "nuchal fold," at the back of each baby's neck. It can sometimes be difficult to make this out conclusively, with three babies crowded into one small area.

Done correctly, NT testing may be able to pinpoint potential Down Syndrome and certain genetic diseases, which could then be verified using other tests.

Ultrasounds

As a triplet mom, you're going to start to feel like a red-carpet celebrity, you'll be having your picture taken so often – or at least, having your womb's photo snapped in the form of increasing ultrasounds as the babies' birth draws nearer.

Early ultrasounds can establish dates, sizes, and viability of the babies, spotting heartbeats and giving important information about how many placentas and sacs there are.

Later ultrasounds keep a close eye on potential trouble situations, like a placenta that's about to separate, cutting off oxygen and nutrients to one or more babies and endangering their lives.

Biophysical profile (BPP)

This isn't a single test, but rather an ultrasound evaluation done late in pregnancy to test and predict the wellbeing of each of the babies. Its results are based on the babies' movement, heart rate, breathing, amniotic fluid volume and more. It's been shown to be effective and useful in triplet pregnancies. A negative result on a BPP – for instance, low amniotic fluid – can lead to a decision to deliver the babies immediately.

Non-stress Test (NST)

Three little hearts beating steadily – you hope, and the NST can help your practitioner make sure everything's still ticking. This test checks to make sure that when they move around, their heartbeats remain steady and strong.

If your babies decide to sleep through the test, your doctor can actually use a buzzer to wake them up.

You may also be advised to drink orange juice or some other healthy source of sugar to ensure that they're lively and active for the test – but don't drink too much, because there are no bathroom breaks allowed: you'll have to lie still for up to an hour while the babies are monitored.

Conditions to watch out for

Lists of symptoms can be alarming to read. It's important to remember that not every pregnant woman experiences every symptom – it can even change from pregnancy to pregnancy. And something which can be a danger sign in one woman may not raise a red flag at all for another. If you are concerned at any time, consult your practitioner, but try not to panic over the number of things that can go wrong.

Remember how many things that have gone right so far – beginning with conceiving after what may have been a long and anxious period of attempting to conceive. Let's hope you never experience any of these problems – or that, if you do, your practitioner is able to intervene and help out in the best way possible.

Bleeding / spotting

Some bleeding is normal, some isn't. How can you tell the difference? The first time you experience any sort of spotting (light bleeding, usually shown as "spots" on your panties), call your practitioner. (If you haven't found a high-risk OB yet, contact your regular family doctor or your fertility specialist).

Depending on your history and where you are in your pregnancy, they'll either have you come into the office, stop by an emergency room, or just reassure you and let you know what trouble signs you should be looking out for. In some cases, when it's believed you're having a threatened miscarriage, you'll have to stay on bed rest for a little while until the spotting or bleeding resolves.

This is one of the most frightening trouble signs during pregnancy because it's associated so closely with miscarriage. But there are so many possible causes of spotting that many, many women experience it at some point and still go on to deliver healthy, happy babies.

Hyperemesis

Throwing up once or twice a day is unpleasant and unhealthy, of course. But if you're still eating and drinking, keeping down most food or water, you're probably going to be fine, as are your babies. Some women even see plenty of morning sickness as a sign of a "strong" pregnancy!

But if you're losing ground nutritionally, dehydrating or your babies are not gaining and growing well as a result of your lack of nutrition, then you are probably suffering from *hyperemesis gravidarum*, a Latin term meaning "excessive vomiting of pregnancy," a description as relevant today as it's ever been.

Hyperemesis may or may not ease as you transition to the second trimester, but in any event, if you can't keep any food down, don't wait! Your triplets need your help to stay fed and happy. In severe cases, hyperemesis may need to be treated on an inpatient basis, so speak to your practitioner as soon as you think you may have a problem.

Breathing difficulties

Some shortness of breath, okay, a lot of shortness of breath, is unfortunately normal with a triplet pregnancy, and can begin very early on, as the babies crowd out your lungs in their competition against you for precious abdomen space.

This is one of those symptoms that you must report to your practitioner, especially if it comes on suddenly.

You may need further tests, like an echocardiogram (EKG) to make sure everything is more-or-less normal – or at least, par for the course with a triplet pregnancy.

Vision problems

Like your skin and your foot size, your eyes may go through natural changes over the course of pregnancy, and you may need an update to your glasses prescription.

Usually, this has to do with the normal changes in your body. But if you start experiencing serious problems, such as temporary loss of vision, sensations of flashing lights, auras, light sensitivity, and blurry vision or spots, these are all warning signs of preeclampsia, and you should contact a medical professional immediately.

Cervical issues

There's no way around it – it's one of the most insulting medical terms out there: *incompetent cervix* (IC). Relax – they're not saying you're incompetent, even though it can feel that way when you first hear the term.

What it means is that, usually based a history of previous miscarriages, or due to shortening of the cervix too early in pregnancy, your doctor is concerned that your cervix – the bottleneck that keeps your uterus safely closed – won't be able to stay shut and hold your babies in tightly enough.

The simple procedure to do this, called *cerclage*, works exactly like you'd think it would: under general, spinal or epidural anesthesia, the doctor enters through the vagina to place stitches around the cervix to ensure that it stays shut as long as it's supposed to.

In a few cases, doctors can opt to enter through the abdomen, in a slightly more complicated procedure. Either way, the stitches then help support the natural muscle of the cervix.

Cerclage is usually done around 14 to 18 weeks as an outpatient procedure. The stitches are removed later on in pregnancy to prevent labor problems. Complications are very, very rare, and many women say the procedure gave them the peace of mind to continue their pregnancy feeling more relaxed and optimistic.

Susan: "I was nervous, but I'm so glad we went with the cerclage. The spinal was quick and didn't hurt much, and afterwards, I didn't feel anything while she did the cerclage. They monitored me in the hospital for about six or seven hours until the anesthesia wore off. There were no complications, and this time I carried to term. This was absolutely the right decision for me."

Pre-eclampsia

Also known as Toxemia and Pregnancy-Induced Hypertension (PIH), this is the big red flag condition that all practitioners will be watching for vigilantly throughout your pregnancy, and it can begin at any point. In your case, it's a special concern: pre-eclampsia develops in half of all triplet pregnancies.

In some cases, bed rest and treatment may alleviate symptoms for a while, but generally, once it begins, pre-eclampsia requires careful monitoring, and may mean a one-way ticket to the delivery room. The big red flags for pre-eclampsia are protein in urine and extremely elevated blood pressure.

This condition is dangerous to both you and your babies, so be watching for specific trouble signs, including changes in vision and headaches. Swelling used to be considered a possible sign of pre-eclampsia, but it's not used for diagnosis anymore. Pre-eclampsia, PIH, and other variations such as HELLP (Hemolysis Elevated Liver enzymes Low Platelet count) syndrome are all dangerous conditions which may not bring any symptoms at all.

That's one big reason why regular doctor check-ups are so important.

Gestational Diabetes

As with some of the other conditions listed here, triplets bring triple the joy but also an increased risk of developing gestational diabetes at some point in your pregnancy. This may be because the larger number of placentas increases your body's resistance to insulin.

If you are diagnosed with gestational diabetes, you'll have to work with your practitioner to create a diabetic diet and perhaps also manage the condition with insulin.

The good news is that gestational diabetes usually goes away once the pregnancy is over, although it's possible that you may have a greater chance of developing it later in life as a result.

Anemia

Anemia is a lack of red blood cells, and it can happen to anyone, at any time; it's not a special pregnancy condition. But you're more vulnerable to anemia when you're pregnant... because you've got more blood than ever before, and sometimes, not enough red blood cells to go around.

Normally, you have about four and a half liters of blood, and in a regular pregnancy, that can go up by nearly one and a half liters. With your doctor's approval, a supplement containing folic acid, iron and vitamin B12 can help prevent anemia during pregnancy, however some supplements – especially ones that contain iron – can be difficult to digest.

Anemia can leave you feeling dizzy and weak – even more so than is normal during pregnancy. You may also look paler than usual or feel your heart beating extra fast. Anemia can affect your baby's growth and development, so this is one of the things you'll be checked for regularly if there are red flags.

Placenta previa

This is literally a "blocking" placenta – it happens when a placenta grows over the cervix, the opening of the uterus. Women with this condition may experience heavy bleeding near the end of the second trimester (or earlier).

Bleeding may start and stop on its own. In single pregnancies, placenta previa usually brings the disappointment of knowing a caesarean delivery lies ahead – however, this probably won't come as such a shock to anyone pregnant with triplets.

Your practitioner may recommend bed rest and will almost certainly tell you not to put anything in your vagina, as well as giving you a list of signs to should watch out for.

TTTS: Info & Tips

Jamie: "My identical triplet boys shared a placenta, so they put me on bed rest at 12 weeks. They had Triplet to Triplet Transfusion [syndrome] and we went to our nearby tertiary center to have the surgery done. All three of my baby boys made it and are healthy! I made it to 34 weeks gestation, and none of them have issues, I am happy to report. Please don't be worried and if you ever have any questions about anything you can feel free to write any of us or message me. Two are home already and my third is a little small but almost ready."

It's usually called "Twin to Twin Transfer Syndrome" (TTTS) because it's most common in twins simply because there are far more twin pregnancies.

In triplets and other multiples beyond twins, what is more accurately called "feto-fetal transfusion syndrome" (FFTS), occurs when blood moves from one baby to another. Essentially, all three babies are competing for resources inside your body, which is why their growth is monitored so closely, but if they share placental circulation, FFTS becomes an extra risk.

The baby losing blood is called the "donor," while the baby receiving the blood is called the "recipient." In the past, the donor baby would ultimately have failed to thrive in utero, and would have died.

For both babies, there are potential health risks, including underdevelopment of the kidneys in the donor and increased blood flow that can cause heart and neurological problems for the recipient.

Today, a "staging" system is used to identify the severity of the FFTS – from Stage I to Stage V. Some interventions are available, from draining amniotic fluid, in relatively minor cases, to laser surgery, for the most severe cases of FFTS. Surgery carries some risk to both fetuses, however, and it's not generally done unless there's no choice.

With the least severe stages, most practitioners take a watchful waiting approach, monitoring carefully once signs emerge to make sure both babies can continue to stay healthy.

Because the causes of TTTS/FFTS are unknown, it's uncertain what you as the mom can do to keep your babies healthy, a situation which can lead to feelings of helplessness. But maintaining your body's healthy growing environment is always important, no matter what else is going on.

Kelly: "Around 18 weeks, my boys starting showing signs of TTTS. I did everything I'd heard of: rested, ate well, and drank tons. No idea what did it, but the TTTS signs disappeared and they're all growing fine now. I'm at 29 weeks, 3 days. Don't let the news scare you too much."

Polyhydramnios

Believe it or not, you can have too much of a good thing – in this case, too much amniotic fluid, the warm liquid that surrounds your babies in their amniotic sac(s). This condition, which is often just known as hydramnios, normally occurs in about 1% of pregnancies, but it's much more common in multiple pregnancies.

Sometimes, it just happens, and in most cases, it's not really known why. However, in a multiple pregnancy, the appearance of excess amniotic fluid around one fetus and not enough around another (oligohydramnios) may be an indication of TTTS, in which case, you'll need to be monitored carefully.

Polyhydramnios is associated with certain neurological problems in babies, and if you experience it, your babies will be checked very carefully at birth. In some cases, excess amniotic fluid can be removed (with a needle, as with amniocentesis) to reduce pressure on your cervix; you may also receive medication to prevent preterm labor.

Most triplet moms can't tell they're developing the condition, because they're already so swollen, and also because it may be accompanied by oligohydramnios in another baby.

Trouble signs of pregnancy

It's impossible for any guide to list every possible complication – and it probably wouldn't be very interesting to read. As with everything in life, there are hundreds of possibilities, and the goal here is not to frighten but to educate moms so they can take an active role in their own healthcare and that of their growing babies, just like you'll do for the next eighteen years (or more).

Early in pregnancy – because there's not really such thing as "early" in a triplet pregnancy – ask your doctor what trouble signs to look out for and when to call.

If it sounds like he or she doesn't want to be disturbed, or if the office staff, nurses and others don't sound like they'll be receptive to your calls at any time, and respect your "gut" instincts, you might want to consider finding a more responsive practice.

General symptoms that should set off alarm bells at any point, in any pregnancy, include:

- Bleeding or – beyond the initial period – spotting, or any blood or staining. Bright red blood is particularly alarming; contact your practitioner immediately and save any pads or cloths you've used to absorb it;
- Vision changes, which could be linked to crucial blood-pressure readings;
- Membrane rupture – a sudden or slow leakage of clear fluid from the uterus;
- Severe stomach pain that doesn't go away when you change position.

Birth

Rachel: "I had a terrific pregnancy. Labor started naturally at 34 weeks, 5 days, and I was rushed into an emergency C-section under general anesthesia because they were coming so quickly. My smallest was not quite four pounds; the biggest was over five! The hospital was super-nice, and let me and each baby stay on past discharge until we could all go home together, when the kiddies reached the 2000g mark."

While it is possible to give birth to triplets vaginally – as women have done throughout history – vaginal birth carries a much higher risk of strangulation, since there are three umbilical cords, as well as with difficult presentations (like breech and shoulder births) that today's obstetricians are in many cases less-qualified than ancient midwives to cope with.

That's because the C-section has become the go-to solution for any complicated obstetric situation, since it's a fairly simple procedure which offers great odds of healthy, happy mom and babies at the end of the day.

Home birth?

Barb: "My biggest disappointment was that that I couldn't have my first choice of practitioner. The midwife I was planning on using told me it's illegal for any healthcare professional to attend to a multiple birth outside of a hospital."

The disappointing reality for many triplet moms is that they'll probably not be having their babies vaginally, let alone at home. In a completely uncomplicated pregnancy, with the babies' positions verified by repeated scans, it is theoretically possible to give birth at home naturally, but in reality, only the world's most experienced midwives would be comfortable going into such a situation.

Though they may initially be disappointed, as the end of pregnancy nears, most moms come to terms with the realities of their situation, and may accept it as the best thing, given their swelling proportions and increasing discomfort, which all drive home the reality of the babies' size and the difficulty of giving birth vaginally three times in a row.

A doula may be an ideal compromise in a hospital situation – a birth aide who can advocate for you before, during and after the C-section surgery, humanizing the experience and easing your homecoming while providing the type of companionship normally offered by a midwife during an uncomplicated vaginal birth.

Find out if there are any doulas practicing locally, and what services they offer to multiple-birth moms.

> Janey: "I originally dreamed of a home birth, but having triplets changes so many things. I was up against a range of issues along the way that most singleton, or even twin, moms just don't have to face. Triplets are way more premature, and way more stress on your body. I had to focus more on what was most important, and less on exactly where and how they would come into the world."

The early birds

It's just a fact of life: almost all triplets, 90%, are born "early," even in a complication-free pregnancy. So prematurity is not going to be listed in the section of "when things go wrong."

Even when everything goes right, your triplets will likely arrive on the scene early than anyone expects.

Patricia, who we met earlier in the book at 31 weeks, knows she'll be delivering within the next three or four weeks, even though she's had an uncomplicated pregnancy so far.

In fact, the mean gestational period (sort of like an average) for triplets is only 31 weeks, so she's already doing better than many, just having carried them this far.

If you start experiencing problems, even 31 weeks may start to seem like an impossible dream. If two or more of the babies share an amniotic sac, there's a greater chance that something can go wrong, and in some cases, the babies will have to be born even earlier to prevent danger.

Additionally, if there's a problem with a placenta, or if you develop preeclampsia, delivering the babies may be the only choice to prevent a life-threatening situation.

Because these babies are born so early, low birth weight is a common complication. This is generally classified as any baby born at less than 5.5 pounds (2,500 grams), but let's face it: 5.5 pounds is a lot of baby when you're carrying three of them in your belly.

For triplets, it's more likely that your babies will be even tinier, and all babies under 3.3 pounds (1,500 grams) have a much higher incidence of complications like mental retardation, cerebral palsy, vision loss, and hearing loss.

One thing you should know is that it appears from lots of research that, unlike in situations of single pregnancies, multiple babies (including triplets) born to older moms don't have an increased risk of complications compared to those born to younger moms.

That's probably because triplets tend to be born to older women who underwent fertility treatment and then received excellent medical care, diet, etc.

Every triplet mom prays for her pregnancy to last as long as possible and her babies to be born as big as possible... regardless of how uncomfortable she feels as a result.

If only there was a way to cross our legs and keep them inside until *we're* good and ready. Still, though we're ultimately not in control, every day that passes and every ounce they gain is a step in the right direction!

Alice: "My pregnancy went very well, actually. No complications, and I carried them to 33 weeks, when I went into labor naturally. They were all high four-pounders, and spent 17, 23 and 36 days in the NICU."

When things go wrong

Triplet moms sometimes get irritated at friends and family who go on and on about the "miracle of birth" when just about everything about their pregnancy and birth experience may fall short of that miraculous idea.

It's understandable that thinking of your sister-in-law's unmedicated, uncomplicated water birth can be painful when facing the prospect of a labor and birth experience complicated by conditions with scary names like malpresentation, vasa praevia, cord prolapse, placental abruption, cord entanglement, and postpartum hemorrhage.

Yet, for all that, even the most hospital-centered birth can indeed be a miracle. Today, we have technology to save even the tiniest preemies, and triplet birth is no longer the scary complication it once was.

You are not alone on this convoluted journey, and understanding some of the potential obstacles along the way can empower you to see through the monitors and medical terminology to the miracle that will someday soon let you hold three incredible babies.

Cord problems

You're pregnant three times over, so that means not one, not two, but three umbilical cords.

Sometimes, the umbilical cord can get one or more babies in trouble, and cause complications even in a single pregnancy – and yes, there's a greater risk of this as well with multiples.

The two most common issues with umbilical cords are tangling in the uterus and being delivered prematurely, before the babies are born. When part of an umbilical cord is delivered before the baby, called cord *prolapse*, it can cut off the baby's vital oxygen and mean an immediate emergency delivery.

Other possible complications, with so many umbilical cords floating around, include knotting, twisting or entanglement of umbilical cords. If all your babies are snug inside their own sacs, the risk of cord problems diminishes significantly.

But if two or more babies share one sac, complications could lead to a diminished blood supply to one or more baby. Some of these issues, diagnosed via ultrasound, may be serious enough to warrant immediate delivery.

Placental abruption

Normally, the placenta is firmly secured to the lining of the uterus. In a standard vaginal delivery, the placenta separates after the baby is born, and slides out as the "afterbirth."

Placental abruption, or abruptio placenta, happens when the placenta begins to separate from the uterus before the babies have been born. The riskiest period is during the third trimester, and this condition can be serious and lead to immediate emergency delivery.

Any signs of an abrupting placenta should be investigated thoroughly – right away – including blood or spotting, especially late in pregnancy, although there isn't always external bleeding. Pain or tenderness in or around the region of your "bump" or back can be another sign, although it's important not to panic, because there are many possible causes of discomfort in these regions.

An ultrasound can usually detect an abruption or (hopefully) put your mind at ease.

Cerebral Palsy

Perhaps as many as 3% of infant triplets are diagnosed with cerebral palsy (CP), a neurological injury which has no known cure. This is probably due to the high rate of prematurity in triplets. Babies born before 32 weeks are twenty times more likely to develop CP than those who go beyond 36 weeks.

CP can develop during pregnancy, birth, or even in the weeks after birth. Because the causes of CP aren't really understood clearly, there's not much you can do to try to prevent it, short of ensuring your pregnancy is as healthy as possible, including diet and hand washing, since certain illnesses during pregnancy may increase your babies' odds of being born with CP.

Misshapen Head

Your uterus is not a big place – even for one baby, by the end of pregnancy, it's hardly an Olympic-sized swimming pool, let alone for three, particularly if there's excess amniotic fluid (polyhydramnios).

If a baby is squashed too tightly at certain crucial stages of development, there's a chance that he or she will develop one of a few conditions, such as plagiocephaly, torticollis, and craniosynostosis (which takes several forms).

These conditions can cause an unusual or even alarming appearance, but are sometimes correctable. Some of the simpler forms of plagiocephaly (also sometimes known as "flat head"), which can affect the alignment of the jaw and teeth, can be corrected with helmets, positioning and exercises.

It's often accompanied by torticollis, or twisted neck, which is also somewhat correctable with physical therapy.

Other conditions, such as craniosynostosis, where the skull bones fuse before the baby's brain is finished growing, are potentially more serious, both in terms of their effect on the baby's appearance and on their potential impact on brain development. Surgery is possible in extreme cases to relieve pressure on the brain and ensure the best possible outcome.

Ongoing sensory issues

Researchers, doctors and parents are now starting to believe that even if multiples escape some of the more obvious and scary diagnoses at birth, they may still be at risk for what are known as "sensory issues" as they grow up.

Sometimes known as Sensory Processing Disorder, these issues can often be confused with mild autism, Asperger's syndrome or ADHD, so it's important to get a correct diagnosis.

Signs that one or more of your babies have a sensory issue may not emerge until their second year, but you may start to see signs early. Small babies may seem very sensitive to touch and perhaps not enjoy being touched or handled. They may also seem to miss hearing certain things or respond in an unusual way to stimuli around them, seem clumsy, particularly irritable or sensitive to their environment.

Once hearing, vision and other problems have been ruled out, it's a good idea to find a specialist who has experience managing sensory processing disorders (SPDs).

What You'll Need for Babies

The great news is that what you need is – not as much as you might think. The bad news is that, with three babies on the way, what you do need, you may need in threes.

But nobody ever said it all has to match – there's no shame in accepting donations from friends or buying the necessities secondhand.

When accepting secondhand items, safety is paramount. Whether it's a crib, swing, car seat or any other baby product, recalls are frequent due to safety concerns.

Search online (http://www.cpsc.gov/en/Recalls/) to check if there has been a recall. If there has, there may still be hope. In many cases, a manufacturer will provide a free retrofitting kit to bring your product up to safety standards. Manufacturer contact information is always included in the recall details.

Necessary Equipment

Car seats

In most areas, you won't be allowed to bring your babies home unless they're in car seats. It's for their own safety, so this is one rule you shouldn't try to get around. If you purchase or receive secondhand car seats, check them carefully.

There should be an expiry date sticker prominently on the seat. All car seats also have a manufacturer sticker with the model number – check online for recalls before using the seat. You can also download user manuals online to be sure that the seats are installed properly. You can also visit a professional car seat installer for extra peace of mind, or some local police departments offer this service free.

Crib(s)

The crib is one area where the Rule of Threes may get to be broken. Many families find they can get by with only a single crib, in fact, and that their triplets enjoy the closeness of sleeping together and, later, of playing together when they wake up.

Sharing a crib, however, may mean that your babies need to move up to toddler beds earlier than they ordinarily would – three in a bed gets crowded fast! But today, it's usually recommended that you take babies from the crib as soon as they're learning to climb. It also goes without saying that, as with any crib, you keep padding and stuffed toys to a minimum. Particularly when there are three wiggly babies, these can lead to suffocation.

Baby carriers

Whether it's a Baby Bjorn or a simple wrap, you'll want baby carriers that can help you carry one baby at a time – or on the front of any adult who's willing to take on a baby for a short while. Use baby carriers to take a walk or just to get things done around the house.

When babies are little, they have to go on your front, and you'll probably find it easier to "wear" them high and tight – as far up on your chest as is comfy for you. Facing outwards may be fun for the baby as it grows older, but it throws their weight forward, away from your body, making it harder on your back and shoulders, so in the early months, it's best to have the baby facing you so you'll both be comfortable.

Don't worry – the baby won't suffocate! If you're worried, just turn their little head to the side for air.

Stroller

This is where many moms of multiples get creative – especially at first, you don't necessarily need a triple stroller, which is great news for your wallet. In the early months, you may be able to get away with putting two babies side-by-side in a single stroller.

Consider borrowing one from a friend until you need to expand the available space a little. So where does the third baby go? Into a baby carrier, once you're feeling up to carrying the weight (if you're not, rope another adult into coming along and strap the baby carrier onto them!). After that, you'll want to go up to a double or triple stroller, but you don't have to break the bank.

Try networking through organizations for multiple parents in your local area before you walk into a store to look at new models.

High Chairs

This is another purchase you can put off for a while. Your babies aren't going to be sitting up and eating solids for a little while. In fact, many parents find it easier to use car seats on the floor to introduce their babies' first solid foods (a misnomer because they're invariably mushy). Line the car seats first with something waterproof, if possible, because they're going to get messy.

Later on, you probably will need high chairs, but these don't have to be fancy and they don't have to match unless you've got the budget for it. Check out garage sales for bargains or ask around your neighborhood to see if anybody has one they're finished with. Because they can take up a lot of space, consider models that fold up for storage.

Another option is a booster seat that straps securely onto a regular kitchen chair and comes with a tray table. Some models of these also fold up when not in use, so you can just push them into the table. These also help later on with the transition to eating straight from the table.

Good-to-have Equipment

This is the whole, huge category of items you may want to have for your babies, but which aren't, strictly speaking, a necessity. Mobiles, baby gyms, walkers (providing they meet updated safety guidelines), bouncers... they're all fun to have.

These are great gift items and also available as hand-me-downs, but be sure you don't take more than you have the space for, especially if it's something your babies won't be using for a while. Certainly, for most of these items, you don't need three.

Then, there's the category of equipment that's "on the line" – most parents do have these things, but you can get by without them to save money or space. Baby bathtubs, for example, take up a lot of space. Consider bath seats instead – these let you wash babies one-handed, you can set them up in the regular tub, and they take up less space when not in use.

Rocking chairs and change tables are two more items in this category. Some moms can't imagine having a baby without one or the other, but they do take up a ton of space and don't come free, either.

Any comfy chair or sofa can be used for feeding babies, and a bed or dresser can be converted instantly, with a waterproof pad, into a change table. A bed may even be safer than a change table if you have three to diaper – safe in the middle, newborns are less likely to roll off, though you still have to keep an eye and a hand out just in case.

In general, don't "stock up" on things your babies cannot use at the moment unless you have a lot of storage space to keep it in. Baby equipment can and will expand to take up every inch available – especially if you have a lot of well-meaning donors! – if you don't stay vigilant and keep the "stuff" in check.

Linens / Clothing List

The list of things you need to dress a newborn is actually pretty short – assuming your house is warm and cozy, your babies won't really care what they're wearing for perhaps five or six years. This list is just a general guideline of the kind of things you might want to consider having on hand.

- Receiving blankets, 8-12 (make sure they're large enough to swaddle; most are too small)
- Baby blankets, 6-9
- Bibs, 8-12
- Fitted crib-sized sheets, 8-10 (this depends on whether you have one or more cribs)
- Quilted pads (plastic one side), or other waterproof pad, 10-12
- Nighties, 3 per baby (nighties are better until the umbilical cord stubs fall off, but this will probably happen before they come home)
- Baby towels (hooded if you like), 4-6, or use regular towels
- Washcloths, 8-12 (soft)
- Sleepers / outfits, 1-3 per baby
- Seasonal: sweaters, bonnets, bunting bags, socks, booties, hats
- Seasonal: snowsuits, if you are expecting winter babies; otherwise, wait until fall to buy these.

Note about clothing: it's almost certain that your babies will be born premature, but you don't know exactly when or how big they'll be. Plus, they may not even all be the same size when they come home. Don't invest in a lot of clothing ahead of time. A few small nighties and/or sleepers per baby will be sufficient until they are home and growing, and then you'll know what sizes you need.

Diapering: Cloth or Disposable?

Some parents are horrified at the thought of using cloth diapers for *three* babies. Others are horrified at the amount of waste that will pile up if they're throwing away disposables for *three* babies.

In either case, there's an investment: with cloth diapers, that comes ahead of time when you stock up on tiny diapers; with disposables, it's ongoing, as you add diapers to your weekly grocery list and then – inevitably – run out midweek and have to make an emergency run.

There's no right answer for every family. With today's washing machines, cloth diapering is easier and more doable than ever before, and if you stock up, you may only have to wash diapers once or twice a week beyond the newborn stage.

And in the long run, you will probably save money with cloth. But it is one extra item on a checklist that will already be very long, so it's understandable that many parents embrace the convenience of throwing diapers away.

If you choose to use cloth diapers, there are lots of groups and forums online that can guide you towards choosing the most convenient option.

Cloth diapers and covers have come a long way since your grandparents' day, and there are sophisticated combinations of diapers, liners and covers that hold everything in while adding a cute and comfortable layer of padding to your babies' bottoms. If you're planning on using disposables, don't stock up on one size; you can buy these when the babies are ready to come home, and by then, you'll have a better idea of what size(s) fit best.

Birth and Beyond

In case you'd hoped that having triplets would get less complicated once they're born – well, not exactly.

But the good news is that your body will ultimately bounce back, and although it might not feel like it at first, you'll have more energy to deal with the specific needs of your new babies.

Complications to watch out for include language and speech delay, cognitive or motor delays, and behavioral problems.

Beyond medical issues, you should also keep in mind the financial, social and emotional repercussions of caring for your sweet little trio.

C-Section Recovery

After six or seven months of feeling awful during pregnancy – get ready for it – you're going to feel even worse.

A C-section is major surgery, there's just no way around it. You'll be unable to pick up your babies, or even laugh or sneeze comfortably, but the good news is the light at the end of the tunnel. Unlike pregnancy, where symptoms seem to intensify, your C-section "symptoms" should get better and better with each passing day, though there may be ups and down and short-term setbacks.

Right after the C-section, you'll probably feel groggy and perhaps nauseous. Over the next few days and weeks, you'll become more conscious of your scar, which at first, may be somewhat shocking in appearance. It should gradually fade, along with the discomfort.

During that time, in addition to the complications of C-section recovery, you will probably also experience "regular" post-partum issues like mood swings, engorged breasts, and vaginal discharge.

Here are a few tips to help you through the first little while after your C-section:

- Support your incision with a pillow, if possible, whenever you cough, sneeze or move around. (Your stitches won't burst, but you'll be more comfortable with a pillow.)
- Drink and drink and drink. This will speed things up in your intestines and get everything back to normal faster.
- Avoid foods that cause gas at first – cabbage, beans, or anything else that could irritate your system.
- Take stairs backwards (going up or down) to ease the pressure on your abdomen.
- Get outside as often as you can – sunlight can help ease postpartum depression.
- Use ice packs to soothe a sore vagina or perineum.

In the NICU

The NICU can be frightening when you're not used to it – unfamiliar sounds, terminology, and behind it all, incubators with the world's tiniest, fragile people.

Most parents of multiples have nothing but good things to say about the staff, particularly the nurses, in the NICUs they've encountered, but there are always exceptions – staff who are abrupt, rude, or just generally abrasive. Remember that bedside manner usually has little relationship with how well they are caring for your babies, although if you have concerns about the treatment they're receiving, be sure to voice these to a sympathetic staff member.

As unfamiliar as the NICU may be, you are your babies' advocate, so start preparing now to help them get better quickly so they can come home soon.

Apnea / Bradycardia

Your babies' internal systems probably won't be as mature as if they'd had the full nine months most babies get to develop, so it's no wonder they have problems sometimes with even the most basic functions – breathing and keeping their little hearts beating.

Often, premature babies stop breathing for a period of time while they're resting or sleeping. In the NICU, babies are monitored so that professionals can respond quickly if a baby isn't breathing. This has usually resolved completely by the time babies comes home, and most parents are relieved to know that this form of apnea is not at all related to SIDS.

Often, following an episode of apnea, a baby may also experience bradycardia, when their heart rate slows, sometimes to under 80 beats per minute. If this happens, nurses and other medical professionals may have to step in again to stimulate the baby's heartbeat.

In general, babies are kept in the NICU until the risk of bradycardia is over, so this has become a rite of passage, sort of a "graduation" milestone from the NICU.

Many parents of triplets and other premature babies have annoyed memories of when their babies were on "brady watch" – observing their babies closely for a period of time, often five days. If a baby "fails" brady watch, he or she will have to stay longer – even if his/her siblings have already gone home.

Nina: "It's so frustrating! He'll go three or four days without a brady, then decide to have one, and that means the five day countdown begins all over again. We are now four days brady-free; I hope he makes it through tomorrow so he can come home at last."

Breastfeeding

Allison: "My milk came in early, I was lucky. All three exclusively breastfed, with no formula at all, for about seven and a half weeks. After that, their demand overtook my supply and I had to supplement with formula."

You can nurse triplets. It's possible, and it's been done before, but let's be honest: it's a lot harder than with one, and no matter what the die-hards say, you'll probably have to supplement at some point.

Don't let that discourage you! Many women who breastfeed, even for a short time, and even if they've supplemented at some point, have said it's a rewarding experience and a lovely way to bond with their babies.

The logistics may seem overwhelming. Two breasts, three babies, crying and hungry. You're going to need professional help. During your pregnancy, make sure you connect with a local breastfeeding expert, either through La Leche League or another organization.

Many lactation consultants are actually certified through the International Lactation Consultant Association, and you can often find these through directories online. Try to find somebody who's helped with multiples before, though you may not find somebody who has triplet experience. Make sure you feel a rapport with whoever you connect with, and that she knows and respects your goals. Whether you are committed to nursing exclusively, or plan to supplement at night, or some other combination of breast milk and formula, she should be prepared to assist you in having the best experience possible.

When breastfeeding any baby, positioning is probably the most important issue, and complicating things in your case is going to be the discomfort following a C-section, plus the complexities of finding a place to put two babies (and finding somewhere safe and comfortable to keep the third while you nurse two at a time).

If possible, most moms suggest you find a way to nurse lying down, especially at first, as this can make all the difference to your comfort level and improve your odds of being able to nurse successfully.

Chances are, your babies won't be able to nurse at first, even if they're healthy, but most NICUs can help moms pump and pass their milk along to the babies.

You'll need to arrange for a breast pump, hopefully one you can borrow, because this can be a big investment. If the NICU staff can help you get hold of one, all the better, because a hospital-quality pump is so much better and more powerful than home models that it can make or break the nursing experience. You'll need to buy brand-new attachments: tubing, breast shields, bottles and bags to collect and store the milk.

Every model of pump requires different accessories, but often these can be purchased together in a kit for your model of pump.

Leah: "The beginning was the hardest because I was sooo tired, busy, sleep deprived. Make sure you eat and drink enough! Whenever I forgot to drink enough water, my milk would drop dramatically."

Kirsten: "Nursing triplets will make you thinner than you can imagine, while eating more than you ever ate before! It takes a ton to feed those kiddos!"

Baby Care: Finding Help

There's no doubt about it – you will need help. Not everybody who offers will be serious, of course, but anybody who's seriously offering should be taken up on the offer.

Of course it's awkward the first time somebody says, "if there's anything I can do…" and you answer, "would you mind picking up some milk for me on your way home?" But most well-meaning people really are happy to be given concrete ways they can help out. Remember to spread the joy around – even the most well-meaning neighbor or colleague may get sick of helping if it seems like they're the only one taking a turn.

Who's going to help?

Keep a clipboard, make a list. Every time someone offers to help, write it down. Try to think of something specific while you've got them there ready, willing, and able.

Turn their "anything" into a once-a-week evening shift to cuddle the babies and carry them around, or an opportunity to bring over a spare lasagna every Monday.

Tap into all areas you can think of: friends, family, church, coworkers. Start broadcasting your needs before you have the babies, if possible. Let everybody know that it's going to be a crazy time, and tell them you could really use all hands on deck for the first few months.

Figure out who you're closest to. You may need some care that you don't feel comfortable asking your husband or partner to do – for example, if you have a best friend, talk to her ahead of time about helping you out in the shower for a couple of weeks as you get better after your C-section.

Friends who have slightly older kids may be a good bet for this type of tasks. Figure out also who you'd be comfortable asking to do menial tasks, like taking out garbage, doing laundry, and cleaning the bathroom. These sometimes fall to the husband or partner, but remember, he's probably going to be exhausted, too, with his hands full of babies every chance he can get.

Don't be disappointed if someone offers to help and then doesn't. There are always going to be a few people who toss out that cheery, "let me know if there's anything I can do!" and then head back into their own lives without giving you a second thought.

If they're good friends or family members, put them on the list for the first birthday party and then forget about them until you're in a saner place.

Others may be great with gifts, and happy to bring stuff, but won't really want to stick around and actually take care of you or the babies. Knowing the strengths and weaknesses of those you're closest to will help prevent disappointment. Even some of the proudest grandparents are not the cuddly, hands-on type… but they may come through with some money for a house cleaner or nanny.

Hiring a professional

If you live far away from most of your family, aren't well-connected within your community, you'll probably want to consider hiring full- or part-time help.

Of course, even if you have a ton of friends and family, you might still want a professional around, taking care of things like cleaning that you might feel awkward requesting from loved ones.

Or maybe, with so many babies, you want somebody experienced to help get them on a schedule and make sure they're being settled into a routine that will work for your family in the long term.

Even families who can't afford it often end up hiring somebody once their triplets come home. This can make a really special "baby gift" from a close friend or relative. Be certain to check the nanny's qualifications, and it's best to find somebody who has experience with multiples if you can.

She doesn't need three arms, but a little experience juggling more than one baby can give her an edge and watching her can help give you the confidence you'll need when you're on your own.

Your Other Kids

If you've got kids already, you're going to need extra hands helping out with them as well. Their routines will need to continue as normally as possible. At the very least, you'll need to make sure mealtimes and bedtimes continue on roughly the same schedule they were on before.

Depending on their age, this may also mean getting others on board to help with getting them to daycare, school, playdates with friends or after-school activities like sports and swimming lessons. Some of these are "fun tasks" that are easy to give away to aunts, uncles, cousins and friends, but make sure you don't write yourself out of the picture altogether.

The triplets are important, of course, but, especially if you were on bed rest during your pregnancy, you need to schedule as much "mom time" as possible with each of your other children once the babies arrive.

Your older children's feelings are far more complex than the little ones, and if they see – at least sometimes – that you're willing to hand over the babies to someone else so you can be with them at a ballet recital, soccer game, their first day of kindergarten, shopping trip to the mall or just at home working on an art project one-on-one, they'll see that they're still a big part of your lives, and probably feel less resentful of their new baby siblings.

Planning Shifts

It sounds like something out of a daycare organization manual, but since that's basically what you'll be running for the next few years, a little organization can't hurt.

Once your babies are home – or before, if you have other kids, it's time to put together a schedule and get everybody helping out, at least until you all start to get into a solid routine.

How you schedule will depend on you, but in some families, it works well to put up an actual, printed schedule somewhere central, like on the fridge, so that anybody coming by can pencil themselves in for something – a meal, a baby-care shift, a walk during the day, a shopping trip.

When will it end? How many weeks or months of meals should you plan for or accept? That's really different for everybody. It depends in part on your own recovery, on your babies' temperaments, and – of course – on when they come home from the hospital.

At some point, you may decide that you don't need as much help, and you're starting to wish more for privacy than for an extra pair of hands around the house.

Keep in mind that some of your helpers may be hurt if you suddenly cut them off, so break it to them gently and let them know that they can continue to stop by, go out for walks, have you over for visits – just not on as rigidly-scheduled a basis as they have been.

Saying Thanks

It's a good idea, perhaps around six months, or – if six months is still too overwhelming – as part of your babies' first birthday celebration, to thank the people who have put so much time, love and energy into caring for your family during those first difficult weeks and months.

You don't have to spend a ton, but giving each person a nice card or framed picture of the triplets can let them know in a more formal way just how grateful you are that they were there for you.

The First Year

Milestones

When they're premature, pretty much everything you've read and heard about milestones – those important "should" dates of the first year of babies' lives – simply goes out the window.

The most important thing to know is that they're only *guidelines*. The second-most important thing is that the order your babies accomplish these milestones is more important than any specific date or timeline.

Here's how practitioners do the "prematurity math": since a typical pregnancy lasts about 40 weeks, milestones are generally calculated from that date. So if a baby is eight weeks premature, that baby isn't expected to start hitting two-week milestones until he or she is eight weeks old.

Triplets born at 30 weeks have at least ten weeks of catching up to do before you should even start sneaking a peek at any list of milestones.

Whatever you do, don't compare your babies, with each other or with others you may see! Sometimes, triplets attain milestones around the same time, which can be extra-cute.

But sometimes, they don't. Perhaps one of the three is at a big size disadvantage, or has other obstacles to overcome. Or, as with any group of three kids, maybe their different personalities mean they'll develop in different ways as they get older. If two of your triplets are identical twins, there's a better chance they will hit certain milestones simultaneously.

Physical Development

Because ages at which babies accomplish different tasks can vary so widely, these are just guidelines. If a baby is showing no signs of attaining a milestone, it's worth following up with a practitioner.

But if, for instance, she's working every minute on rolling over and it's clear she'll get there soon – don't panic; just let her work it out in her own good time.

Because many triplets have developmental issues, occasionally you'll need extra help, from an occupational therapist or another specialist, to help one or more baby reach a milestone.

Remember to do the prematurity math and add the number of weeks early your babies were born!

- 1-3 months, smile, raise head and gain head strength on tummy, track objects with eyes, grabs at dangling toys
- 4-6 months, roll over, laugh, grab objects, gain complete head control, leg strength,

may enjoy being held to stand, and begin to sit

- 7-9 months, sit without support, may begin to crawl or move in some other way, clap and play simple games like "peekaboo," may learn to pull to a standing position, begin self-feeding
- 10-12 months, acquire greater control when self-feeding, including "pincer grasp," move around in some way, point to "ask" for objects, play with toys and may be starting to walk.

How you can help:

You can help your babies' physical development by giving each baby enough "tummy time" and other opportunities for independent play throughout the day.

While at first, you may be carrying them constantly, later on in the first year, you'll want to let them entertain themselves, and each other. But you'll need to balance that with the difficult job of giving each baby physical one-on-one time with you or their other parent for lifting, swinging, dancing and other fun physical activities.

Language

Another common area of concern is language development, where twins and higher-order multiples are often slightly behind their singleton peers. You may have heard that multiples develop their own language among themselves, and this may be one reason they're not as quick to pick up the spoken language of the adults around them; they're too busy having fun among themselves!

Remember to do the prematurity math and add the number of weeks early your babies were born!

- Under 1 month, babies learn to recognize familiar voices and use the same cry for all needs.
- 1-4 months, react to sounds by blinking or another response, and begin to "talk" with cooing sounds
- 5-6 months, recognize their name and babble with repeated sounds like "ma-ma"
- 7-9 months, understand facial expressions and some words, like "no." May repeat or mimic words and wave "bye-bye."
- 10-12 months, understand parent names and identify parents, and perhaps use the names correctly.

How you can help:

You can help your babies' language development by talking and singing to them often, and insisting that other caregivers do so as well.

From their very earliest days, babies might not be able to understand, but they thrive from social contact and from hearing language constantly. But turn off the TV! The eye contact that comes along with true social contact is far more valuable for teaching language skills than the impersonal box sitting in the corner.

Out and About

First Outings

If you were able to network with experienced multiple mommies during your pregnancy, you may have been amazed with the ease and grace with which they bundle up babies, bottles, blankets, car seats, baby carriers, changing pads, diapers and more for each and every outing. Maybe you thought you could never do all that yourself... but you will.

Within a couple of months, you will be that experienced multiple mommy, juggling babies and all their stuff with a practiced ease. If only you could see a picture of yourself one year from today, you'd be amazed!

What to Pack

First of all, even though they sell special diaper bags for twins and triplets, you might not need one. In fact, you might not need a special diaper bag at all. Some have special features like a changing pad and wet bag, but any waterproof pad and zippered baggie can substitute for these.

What you need is a big, sturdy bag that can hold lots of stuff – but not necessarily triple the stuff of a single baby. Sure, you'll need extra diapers, but depending on how long you're going out for, probably not three times the quantity.

Here's what you should include in your diaper bag:

- Hand sanitizer
- Change of clothing – in the summer, this can be as simple as a onesie per baby. In the winter, you'll need warmer clothes, extra socks, and more.
- Extra pacifiers in a zippered baggie if any of the babies use them.
- Burp cloths / extra blankets (at least 3)
- Tissues, lots and lots. Consider also bringing a few paper towels prefolded in a zipper baggie.
- Feeding supplies – bottles, bibs, bottled water and premeasured formula packets (measure it yourself at home into zippered baggies to save money)
- Antibacterial ointment, Band-Aids, wipes, and a few other "emergency" supplies.
- Any medications any of the babies need regularly.
- Later on, you'll add solid-food snacks to the bag, including containers of "O" cereals, raisins and other healthy finger foods.
- Grown-up supplies: keys, wallet
- Business card, phone number sticker or some other form of ID (helps get your bag back if you lose it)

You'll notice that diapers aren't on this list. That's because it's best to keep them separate, in an extra-large zipper bag, inside your main diaper bag. Here's what goes in there:

- Diapers – at least six.
- Wipes (a travel-sized package)
- Diaper cream if you use it
- Changing pad
- Hand sanitizer (helpful to have a small bottle inside this bag as well as the one in your "main" diaper bag)
- Doggie bags – these are plastic bags sold in a compact dispenser. Meant for dog walkers, they're the perfect way to ensure that bags stay intact and convenient to tote home (or dispose of) anything messy!

Bring Help

The first few times you venture out, don't go it alone. Even if it's just your husband or partner, even if you're just going around the block, bring along another grownup.

Plan a short outing the first time, and maybe venture a little farther each time – maybe a corner grocery store, a park a few blocks away, or a coffee shop just across the street. If you're still sore from the C-section, you may need another person to wear a baby carrier with one of the babies until you're ready to do it yourself.

It's also useful to have another pair of hands, and to have somebody who can wait outside while you run in and buy a basket of strawberries, a cup of coffee or just push an older child on a swing.

Music / Activity / Playgroups / Playdates

Here's the fun part of life with babies – or at least, it can be fun. Don't start too early – before your babies are old enough to appreciate what's going on! – and don't try to keep up with what other mothers you know are doing.

It really can be as simple as choosing activities that are fun for you and for the babies... and dropping any that aren't.

It's possible to save money on programs in a few different ways. Playdates and playgroups can be free, which is always a plus. If you join any kind of music or activity program, make sure you ask if there's a discount for multiple babies in the same family, and try to find programs that do offer this.

You may also qualify for discounts on certain recreation programs offered by your local area – try to network with other multiple moms to find out what deals are out there.

When you go to check out a class, it's a good idea to bring along a second person, either a friend, family member or a paid caregiver, just to make sure you can give each baby enough attention, or to whisk one away for diapering, if need be.

Just a tip: while you're out having fun with other babies and moms, make sure you don't start talking milestones. Despite what the calendar says, for the first few years, your babies probably aren't going to be doing the same things as other babies their age.

Sleep

Katie: *"Sleep when the babies sleep. Ha ha ha."*

Getting any baby onto a consistent sleep schedule is one of the biggest challenges of the first year. The main thing is doing what you can to help them understand the difference between day and night.

If you keep all the lights blazing and the TV on 24/7, they won't want to settle down at the end of the day.

But if you give them a chance to see that evening is coming, it will gradually become easier as the daily routine becomes familiar.

Create bedtime rituals. This will probably feel strange at first, especially since you know the babies have no intention of dropping off to sleep.

Give them a warm bath if you can (or just brush their hair or do some other soothing routine), put them in PJs, read a story, wipe their gums (or teeth, when they get them), and cuddle them before kissing them and saying goodnight.

Your sleep is important, too. If your babies are bottle-fed, or if you're supplementing with bottles, consider having someone come in to take over for at least a few nights each week.

This may have to be a professional, if you can afford it. By removing yourself from the babies for a few hours, you'll be able to greet them a little more refreshed in the morning.

Therapy

Dawn: *"I was so scared when they said the girls would need ongoing physical therapy. But now we've seen things we only dreamed of when they were born. It's such a miracle seeing them improving and growing and gaining new skills almost every week. It's been amazing, and I feel like we're all part of a team – me, my husband, the girls and our therapists together."*

It's just a reality with preemie babies: one or more of your triplets may need regular therapy sessions. It may be physical therapy, speech-language therapy or other types of intervention to help get everything on track developmentally.

Therapy can be an unwanted outing, but remember that early intervention is now considered the key to language, physical and even emotional development.

Consistency is the most important thing in any kind of therapy for kids – ensuring as much continuity as possible can help your babies make progress quicker.

It's best if they can have the same therapist in the same setting each time, and to continue for an extended period rather than receiving treatment in smaller "blocks." However, in some cases, therapy is only available for a short time – and especially on a limited budget, some is better than none.

With any type of therapist, ask questions to find out what the goals of therapy are. You can become an active participant, as well, by finding out how you can reinforce the therapeutic activities in the home setting, preferably in a casual way that you can incorporate into regular play, social and later, mealtimes.

Feeding: Introducing Solids

You'll want to wait to introduce solids until everything has been okayed by the babies doctor. They should be well beyond any preemie digestive issues, so the regular feeding schedule doesn't apply in your situation.

They should at least be sitting up well and showing an interest in putting things in their mouths before you begin.

Because each baby develops differently, one or two babies may reach this stage before their siblings. You don't have to wait – babies who are ready, willing and able to eat (once their doctor gives them the green light) should be able to start.

You should also check with the doctor to find out if there are any potential concerns with allergies and/or choking, and to find out what his or her opinion is on introducing potentially-allergic foods.

For single babies, the first "solid" foods are usually rather mushy. But there's no law that says you have to spoon-feed each baby. If you delay introducing solids by a few weeks, your babies may have better hand control and be ready to start feeding themselves – a big boon for moms with not nearly enough arms to spoon-feed three babies.

Instead of rice cereal, you may be able to line your babies up in car seats (with bibs) and hand each one a rice cake instead. Later on, bring them to the table – but don't expect food to stay on the table. Introducing cooked whole peas, beans or carrots is another way of avoiding having to spoon-feed the babies all by yourself.

The perennial mom favorite "O" cereals are also great to introduce grains into their diet, as well as toast or other types of crackers. Ask your doctor not only for more information about what order to introduce solids but for help finding alternatives that they can feed themselves.

Whatever your babies are nibbling on, it's going to make a mess. In the warmer months, some moms choose to leave their babies shirtless for their earliest meals because it saves having to wash whatever they're wearing.

Remember to entertain the babies while they eat by singing or reading a story, and do what you can to make mealtimes light and fun.

Don't leave them alone, even with tiny finger foods, even for a second. Choking is very common in the first weeks and even months of self-feeding, and it doesn't take long for a rice cake or piece of toast to become an unmanageable soggy wad that a baby can't swallow.

Con(tra)ception

It happened once, it could happen again. Even if you had to go to extreme measures to conceive this time around, that doesn't mean there's no chance of conceiving again spontaneously. Most doctors and practitioners recommend waiting a while after any "high-risk" pregnancy, especially if there were complications.

How long to wait can vary, but most triplet parents find they have their hands full enough without even thinking about having another baby anytime soon.

Most doctors discuss contraception at the six-week "all-clear" checkup, when they make sure your body has gone back to normal and okay you to start having sex again. It may not take place exactly at six weeks, depending on the circumstances of your birth.

And if your babies are still in the hospital at that point, you may not have an opportunity to be intimate anytime in the foreseeable future. Still, the day will come when you want to have a little intimate fun... make sure you're ready.

The two most commonly-offered forms of birth control postpartum are the Pill and a hormone-enhanced IUD.

There are advantages and disadvantages to each method.

Many women like the control the Pill gives them, adjusting the dose as necessary, but an IUD offers a hands-off approach (nothing to forget every day!) and nearly-guaranteed effectiveness for up to five years.

Whatever form of contraception you choose, remember to find out how long you have to use a backup method before its effectiveness kicks in – for the Pill, this may be the entire first month, and for an IUD, it can vary.

Happy Birthday, Babies!

You did it! You made it through the first year, which of course includes the trying months leading up to the babies' birth.

Pat yourself on the back, pour yourself a drink, book yourself a babysitter. However you want to celebrate is just fine!

You don't have to do anything too splashy for a first birthday party, at any time of year – lots of places rent party rooms, but sometimes, it's overkill for three babies who still don't really know what's going on them. This party is more for you and the bigger people in your triplets' lives than it is for them, although you'll want to take lots of pictures to prove you went all out in celebrating.

If it's a summertime birthday, try to celebrate outdoors – make sure you recruit someone else to make sure the babies don't get into trouble while you're running around spending time with guests and taking care of food.

Better yet, designate someone else to take care of food and you can relax and spend time with the people you love who really haven't gotten a lot of attention over the last year!

You've done it: you made it through a triplet pregnancy, and back again to where you started –

with three more children to make your life so much more interesting than it ever was before.

You have overcome the challenges, you've probably cried an ocean and hopefully laughed just as much, and you also realize there are many more hurdles still to come.

Today, your triplets have reached an incredible milestone; may the years ahead be just as rewarding as the last year and nine months (give or take) and may you continue to learn and grow for a lifetime, together with your little ones.

Triplet Trivia

Did you know...

- Scrooge McDuck's nephews, Huey, Dewey and Louie are identical (BBB) triplets.
- Psychologist Elizabeth Kubler-Ross, who first created the idea of stages of grief, was an identical triplet.
- A 1980 People Magazine story told of three men, Robert Shafran, Eddy Galland, and David Kellman, who became "overnight triplets" – they were separated for adoption at birth and reunited at the age of 19 through a series of incredible coincidences.
- The Del Rubio Triplets were popular nightclub singers in the 1950s, and following their rediscovery in 1985, appeared in many television shows during the 1980s.
- In the 2002 movie, *Minority Report*, detectives of the future solve crimes before they happen thanks to "precog" psychic triplets Agatha, Arthur and Dashiell (all named after mystery writers).
- *Playboy* playmates Nicole, Erica and Jaclyn Dahm created a sensation when they decided to all become pregnant at the same time in

2009 (they were actually the second set of triplets to be featured in the magazine). None of their babies were multiples.

- Lady Gaga's music video *Paparazzi* featured the Landeberg Triplets from Sweden, who also appeared in the VH1 reality show, "Daisy of Love."

- In the 2001 film *Harry Potter and the Philosopher's Stone*, the infant Harry was actually played by triplets, letting the film crew swap in a fresh baby if one started to fuss. If only it was that easy in real life with triplets!

- In February, 2014, Kimberly Fugate of Mississippi, expecting triplets, gave birth to identical *quadruplet* daughters, an event of "almost incalculable" odds, according to her medical team. The fourth baby had been hiding behind her sisters on every single prenatal ultrasound!

More Great Reading

When You're Expecting Twins, Triplets, or Quads: Proven Guidelines for a Healthy Multiple Pregnancy, by Barbara Luke (Author) , Tamara Eberlein (Author)

I Sleep at Red Lights: A true story of life after triplets, by Bruce Stockler

Magical Multiple Moments: Parents of Multiples Share Stories and Advice on Raising Happy, Healthy Twins, by Julie Gillespie

Triplets? Relax!: Tips to Guide You Through the First Year, Sanity Intact, by Victoria Adams

You're All My Favorites Board book by Sam McBratney (Author), Anita Jeram (Illustrator)

The Baby Bump: Triplets Edition, by Carley Roney

The Everything Twins, Triplets and More Book, by Pamela Fierro

From the Author

Now that you have finished this book, please consider recommending it in a review.

Reviews are the best way readers evaluate and discover great new books and I would truly appreciate it. You can post a review here:

www.amazon.com/author/ntgore

Thank you very much!

Back Cover:

Triplet pregnancy is unique, and so are the effects of it on your body, mind, family, and finances. Enjoy the wisdom and insightful experience of actual triplet moms, learn about common medical complications and typical issues, and prepare for and welcome your triplets with confidence with many useful, practical tips!

Topics Include:

- The Joy of Triplets
- First Steps and Preparation
- Considering Selective Reduction
- Medical Complications and Health Issues
- Your Options for Birth
- Triplet Development
- The First Year of Your Triplets
- Sleeping and Eating
- Triplet Trivia
- And much more...